THE INCREDIBLE HEALING NEEDLES

A non-technical explanation of the ancient Chinese science of acupuncture, how it works, the techniques it employs, and its therapeutic significance in the modern world.

By the same authors
ACUPUNCTURE HANDBOOK
FIRST-AID AT YOUR FINGERTIPS
THE FIVE ELEMENTS OF ACUPUNCTURE AND CHINESE MASSAGE
JUDO REVIVAL POINTS, ATHLETES' POINTS AND POSTURE
THE LAWSON-WOOD MULTI-LINGUAL ATLAS OF ACUPUNCTURE
GLOWING HEALTH THROUGH DIET AND POSTURE

THE INCREDIBLE HEALING NEEDLES

A Layman's Guide to Chinese Acupuncture

by

DENIS LAWSON-WOOD F.Ac.A.
&
JOYCE LAWSON-WOOD

NATURE'S WAY

SAMUEL WEISER INC.
734 Broadway, New York, N.Y.10003

First published 1974
Second Impression 1975

ISBN 0 87728 298 6

Typeset in Great Britain by
Specialised Offset Services Limited, Liverpool
and printed and bound by Weatherby Woolnough Limited,
Sanders Road, Wellingborough, Northants.

CONTENTS

CONTENTS

Chapter

PREFACE

Up to 1959 Chinese Acupuncture as a method of healing the sick was almost unknown in Great Britain, but that year the first book on acupuncture ever to be published in the English language appeared. It was entitled *Chinese System of Healing* and was written by the authors of this book. The next year the Acupuncture Association was founded, and a lecture series to train practitioners was started.

During the early years of the Acupuncture Association the relatively small group of researchers, practitioners and students had to cope with many difficulties and obstacles which included ridicule, disbelief, and even organized opposition.

By the early 1970s not only had the Association become well established under the presidency of Sidney Rose-Neil, F.Ac.A., it was also recognized as having its membership made up of the leading and most highly qualified practitioners of acupuncture in Great Britain.

Something else then happened to focus world attention on acupuncture. In the Far East such amazing technical advances were being made that it was possible for acupuncture to be used as the only anaesthetic for even major surgical operations.

It now has to be acknowledged that acupuncture cannot be lightly dismissed as charlatanry, mumbo-jumbo, or faith-healing, but must be accepted as a highly advanced therapy. Publicity has been given on such a wide scale through press, radio, and TV, that more and more people are asking all sorts of questions: What is acupuncture? How does it work? Will it cure me?

To answer some of the many questions and to explain in simple terms what it is all about, and where it fits in to the general medical pattern of our times, this book has been written.

CHAPTER ONE

THE NEI CHING

The oldest medical book in existence was, according to some authorities, written about 4,500 years ago, some date it even earlier. A definite date cannot be given for the book, known as the *Nei Ching Su Wen*, though it is generally accepted by scholars that it was written by the Chinese Emperor Huangti, who reigned from 2696 to 2598 B.C.

It is difficult for us in the present day, when affairs of State are so many and burdensome, to imagine a time when a ruler could himself have enough time, knowledge or interest to feel so intimately and personally concerned with the health and welfare of his subjects to write a book.

The Yellow Emperor's classic of internal medicine (the *Nei Ching*) is, by western standards, one of the most remarkable medical books ever written. It is in the form of recorded conversations between the Yellow Emperor Huangti and his minister Ch'i Pai. The Emperor asks for explanations about diseases, their causes, and the various methods of treatment in use at that time: in particular he asks about the efficacy of acupuncture. Ch'i Pai gives detailed and learned answers.

Right down to the present day this early medical treatise has been looked upon by the Chinese as the basis of their native medicine. Although many commentaries upon the *Nei Ching* have been compiled, and many other medical works have been written, this classic of internal medicine is *the* ultimate authority.

A REMARKABLE WORK

There are a good many reasons why, to us in the West, the *Nei Ching* seems such a remarkable work.

In the first place we cannot help noting this fact; when the *Nei Ching* was written, acupuncture was already well established as a healing method. One of the reasons for writing the book was to have permanent written records of whatever had been experimentally proven over the years to be valid and best. We have to conclude, therefore, that the acupuncture points on the human body had been discovered and plotted long before. We do not consider it to be an exaggeration to claim that the knowledge of acupuncture must be at least five thousand years old. When we explain later on what the acupuncture points are, it will be appreciated that the ancients had knowledge and means of investigation far beyond anything so far attained by western science.

NO REFERENCE TO SURGERY

A second feature we cannot help noticing is that the *Nei Ching* contains practically no reference at all to surgery. This, however, does not mean that there were no surgeons: indeed, according to tradition, there had been several eminent surgeons whose achievements equalled, if not surpassed, anything accomplished at the present time. For example, Pien Ch'iao, (second century B.C.) is reputed to have had such profound knowledge of anaesthesia, and used it so skilfully, that he could carry out major operations quite painlessly. It is even recorded that he was able to exchange the hearts of two patients, and the operation was successful: but, alas, he did not leave any written record of his anaesthetic technique.

It is not known for certain exactly what methods of anaesthesia were used because, unfortunately, the writings of another surgeon and authority on anaesthesia, Hua T'o, were destroyed. In the light of present day 're-discovery' of acupuncture as an effective anaesthetic, it would not be altogether surprising if acupuncture were so used by the ancients.

That surgery is scarcely mentioned in the *Nei Ching* is accounted for by the fact that, in those days, there was so little call for surgery because medical treatment was basically preventive, and diseases were not allowed to develop to the point where operations were necessary. A surgeon was looked upon as belonging to a very inferior class of medical practitioners, who had neither the knowledge nor skill to maintain the good health of his patients. From the patient's point of view, having an operation had no prestige-value, but rather was it a matter for shame.

A DIFFERENT ATTITUDE

To a western practitioner the *Nei Ching* reveals yet another astonishing feature, namely: from the writings, illustrations and diagrams, the ancients did not appear to have the same detailed knowledge of anatomy that we enjoy in the West today. Yet in spite of *appearances* to the contrary we cannot believe that the ancients did not know their anatomy and physiology; indeed it is probable that their knowledge was at least equal to our own. However, their orientation and attitude to life differed from ours; their values and focus of attention were concerned with the laws of nature and their manifestations, rather than the relatively unimportant structural details of anatomy.

Medicine was not a science nor an art on its own, neatly partitioned off from other sciences and arts, but an integral part of their religion and philosophy. Thus, in the *Nei Ching*, we come across philosophical tenets, moral issues, and ethical precepts discussed together with disease and sickness symptoms, all as parts of a greater concept; Way of Life.

CHAPTER TWO

WAY OF LIFE

The traditional concept of Tao, the Way, is so foreign to present-day westerners that it is not surprising to find acupuncture (and more or less all far-eastern medicine) has been looked upon as superstition and quackery. It is not easy for any westerner to understand the far eastern outlook sufficiently to enable him to think habitually in the eastern way. It can be done. In our view, although a western scientifically trained and oriented medical practitioner might achieve a certain amount of technical 'know-how' he will not be able to become a true physician or healer in the highest traditional sense unless and until he makes a serious attempt to understand and put into practice the Principles of the Way of Life expounded in the *Nei Ching*.

It will not be at all easy for the desirable Way of Life to come about because, nowadays, people do not consult a doctor until they are ill; whereas, ideally, one's physician should be regularly visited for advice and guidance in maintaining a high degree of good health. Western doctors are not trained to be guardians of health. A doctor's livelihood depends upon a regular and sufficient supply of sick people requiring medication of one kind or another. Added to this, of course, is the huge commercial interest in drug manufacture – it would be 'bad business' if too many people were healthy and did not need prescriptions.

DISOBEDIENCE OF LAWS

The consideration of medicine as part of a larger unity which includes philosophy, ethics, religion, etc., has not been confined to the Far East. We have, for example, many instances on record in the Old Testament of sicknesses and visitations resulting from disregard of or deliberate disobedience of Laws made known by religious leaders. In both Judaism and early Christianity practising medicine and healing was part of the priestly function. The separation of medicine, and its being set up as an independent science is, in the estimation of many, a definitely retrograde step, no matter in what part of the world it happens.

The conversation between Huangti and Ch'i Pai opens with the emperor asking why, in the old days, people lived to be 140 years old and did not suffer diseases, but now they live to only half that age and suffer all manner of sicknesses and pains.

Ch'i Pai's answer, expressed very simply, amounts to this: In the old days people lived in harmony with the Laws of Nature, obeying them and not going against them.

The Way of Life to be followed, or the Laws of Nature to be observed are primarily those appropriate to an uncomplicated agricultural community, or to simple nomadic peoples. A modern industrialized community would find it well nigh impossible to follow *all* the precepts: nevertheless there are many basic natural laws, cycles and rhythms with which we would do well to co-operate instead of disregard.

CYCLES AND RHYTHMS

In order to give successful acupuncture treatment of the best quality the practitioner *must* know quite a lot about natural cycles and rhythms, and he must know how to use them to advantage. Obviously his patients do not need anything like the same depth and range of knowledge; but, if they are to benefit from acupuncture treatment to the fullest possible extent, it is advantageous to have some understanding, enough to be able to carry out instructions intelligently.

We live in a world of constant change. All, however, is not haphazard and mere chance; there are orderly patterns of change. There is the Solar Cycle which gives us the seasons: there is the Day and Night rhythm also. The moon plays a very important part too: not only does the moon give us the high and low tides of the sea, but the moon also regulates ebb and flow of other fluids and forms of energy.

In common with many other nations the Chinese divide their year into lunar months. As a lunar month is only twenty-eight days (instead of thirty or thirty-one) an extra month has to be added seven times in nineteen years. One can become accustomed to thinking in moons and moon phases.

It is obvious that farmers have to follow the seasons: it is almost too obvious to mention that if one plants or sows seeds in autumn which should be planted or sown in spring there could be no crop at all, or only a very poor one!

Any farmer, the world over, knows that some routine activities should be carried out during a waxing moon, others during a waning moon. Some, though not all, growers know that apples for immediate consumption are best picked during a moon's second quarter; while if wanted for storage they will best be gathered during the fourth quarter.

Correspondingly there are best and proper times and seasons for human activities. There are proper times for waking and for sleeping, for working and resting, eating and drinking; indeed for all the natural human activities and functions. This does not mean that one ought to live 'by numbers' as automatons or robots. Far from it: there is enough flexibility to allow for an infinite variety of individual choice and self-expression. Life would be dull if we were all too alike.

The flexibility is always within certain limits which cannot be overstepped without disorganization or imbalance of some sort resulting. Living in one-ness, or in harmony with nature means that the human activities are in harmonious balance and all the body changes and so on are in correct accord with the Laws of Nature.

Now that we have come to the idea of 'balance' it seems appropriate to introduce two words which we cannot do without in acupuncture: Yang and Yin.

These two forces, urges, or energies when in proper balance, and when complementing and supplementing one another, result in health: but, when unbalanced, conflicting, and disorganized, they manifest as disease.

CHAPTER THREE

YANG AND YIN

The two Chinese words, Yang and Yin, do duty for many English words. In English we have no one pair of opposites to translate all that is implied by the words Yang and Yin. They are labels for ideas or concepts which we have to talk around to try to show what notions are included – but however long the list we give, there will always be more one could add.

In acupuncture one talks about Yang energy and Yin energy: Yang states and conditions, Yin states and conditions: Yang treatments, Yin treatments, and so on endlessly. The principles are, nevertheless, extremely simple; and it should not be difficult for the reader to grasp the general ideas involved.

In nature things *happen*. That is to say, there is a 'going-on' all the time – ceaseless change. There is a patterning to this happening, which we can exemplify in the rhythmic changes of 'day and night', 'desire and satisfaction', 'activity and repose'. Everywhere in nature one sees that it is as if there are two forces at work in dynamic interplay: Light and Shadow, Male and Female, Up-Down, Heat-Cold, Heavy-Light, Compression-Expansion, Concentration-Dispersion, Attraction-Repulsion, etc.

This duality appears universal at every level of existence. These two forces are not separate, independent forces, but rather are they the two poles of a Unitary Power – as if they were the Right and Left Hand of One.

The legendary Philosopher-Emperor Fu Hsi based his formulation of philosophy on the Unitary Principle: All beings, things, circumstances and phenomena are manifestations of the dynamic interplay or balancings of the two poles, Yin and Yang, in infinitely variable complex aggregates.

We prefer to avoid, wherever possible, the use of the terms 'positive' and 'negative' when describing Yang and Yin, because to so many people nurtured in western cultural tradition these terms seem almost inseparably linked with an idea of *values*, 'positive' being thought of as better than 'negative'.

BOTH POLES OF EQUAL VALUE

In the Chinese tradition it is accepted as self-evident that one pole could not exist without the other: both poles are essential and, therefore, basically of equal value. As it is written in the *Tao Teh Ching*, 'The ten thousand creatures cannot turn their backs to the shade without having the sun on their bellies'.

Yang is the name given to the polarity whose force acts centripetally: that is *inwards* towards a centre. If we look at the symbol often used to represent Yang we shall get a very clear idea of what is meant. The symbol shows a circle with four arrows drawn from inside the circumference pointing towards the centre. Yang is seen to label the force of compression, solidifying, holding together, organizing, integrating, densifying, making heavier in weight, etc. In acupuncture the

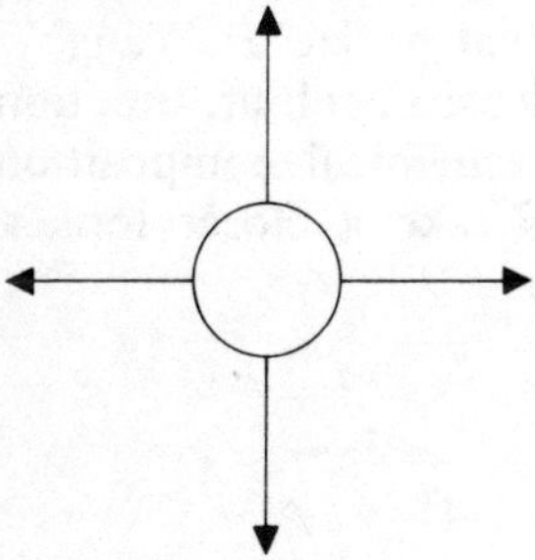
SYMBOL FOR YIN

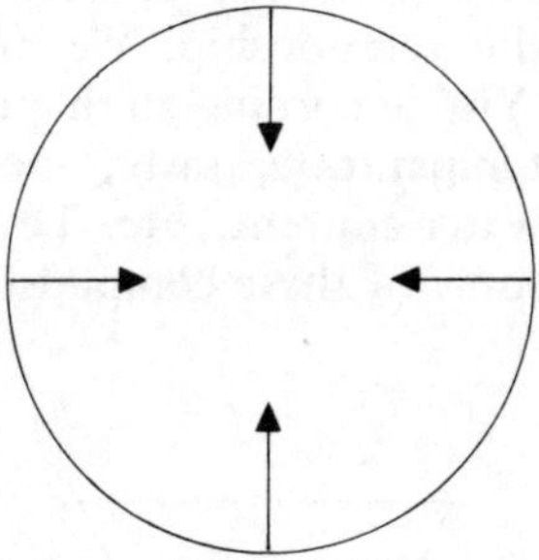
SYMBOL FOR YANG

life-energy flowing through man is labelled Yang when it is flowing in the direction Heaven to Earth.

Yin is represented symbolically by a dot or very small circle with four arrows pointing *outwards*, away from the centre; showing that Yin represents the *centrifugal* force of expansion, loosening, disorganizing, disintegrating, dispersing, making lighter in weight. In acupuncture the life-energy flowing through man is labelled Yin when it is flowing in the direction Earth to Heaven.

It will now be readily understood that just as nothing is 'absolutely long' nor 'absolutely fast . . . hot . . . heavy . . .' etc., so too nothing is wholly nor absolutely Yin or Yang. Yin or Yang beings, things and circumstances are only characterized as Yin or Yang *relatively*. The continued existence of anything is dependent upon the continuance of its own peculiar and characteristic Yang-Yin relative proportions. Again, quoting from the *Tao Teh Ching*: 'On the blending of the breaths their harmony depends.'

Something is only Yang or Yin in relation to

something else. There are many ways of assessing the relationship. We may categorize as 'Yang' or 'Yin' according to shape, density, colour, function, temperature, taste, speed, chemical composition, water-content, etc. Let us take a closer look at some of these comparisons.

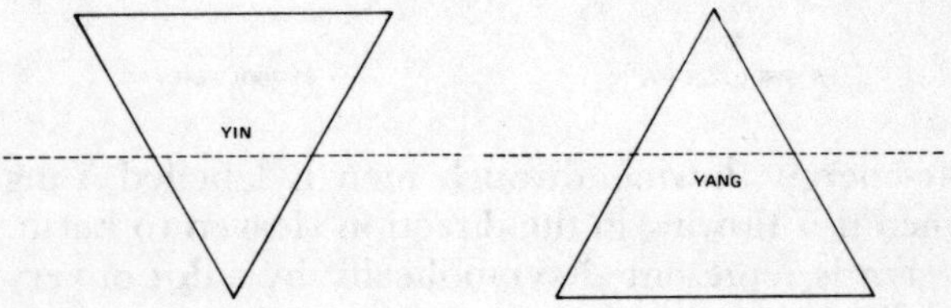

Shape. In general the taller relative to width is the more Yin: the broader and flatter relative to height the more Yang. In the case of triangles, cones, pyramids and so on one assesses which force is dominant by asking: Where is the greater bulk, above or below? Near centre or near periphery? This may be well illustrated by asking, Which, according to shape, is the more Yang, a strawberry or a pear? We must be careful not to be misled by the fact that both these fruits hang from a stalk. The stalk end is nearer the plant centre. Therefore a strawberry will be considered more Yang than a pear. A strawberry is also looked upon as more Yang on account of its colour and on account of mineral content.

Density. In our diagram we represent weight/

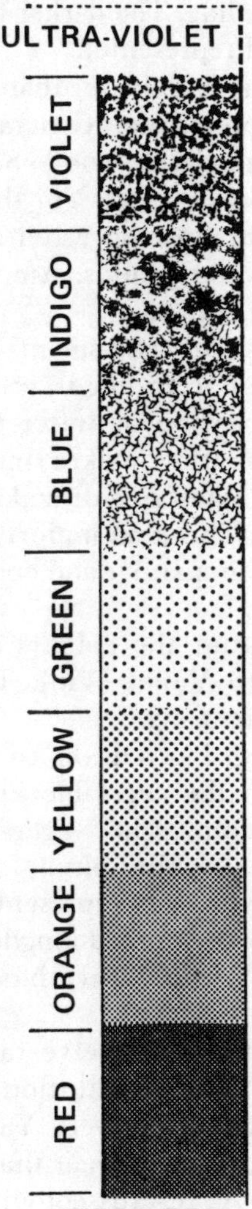
ULTRA-VIOLET
VIOLET
INDIGO
BLUE
GREEN
YELLOW
ORANGE
RED
INFRA-RED

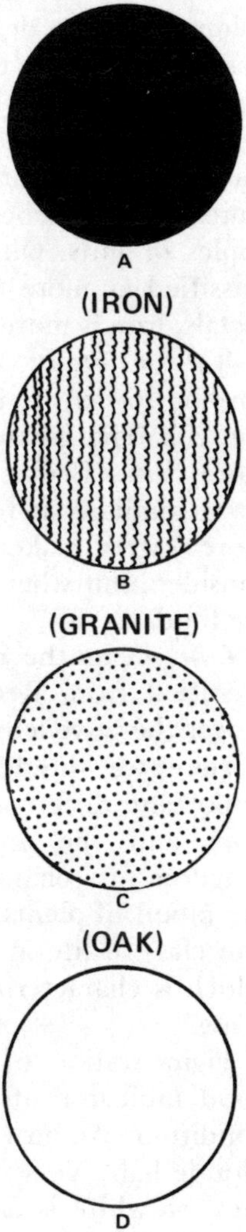
A
(IRON)
B
(GRANITE)
C
(OAK)
D
(CORK)

volume ratio by degrees of shading. The darker the shading the denser the material represented.

All other things being equal, **A** is denser than **B**, **C** and **D**, and therefore more Yang. Generally speaking, metals are more Yang than wood. Soft fruits, like gooseberries, would be more Yin than apples or nuts. Oily fluids that float on water are classified as more Yin than watery fluids. Among metals, iron is more Yang than copper.

Water-Content. Very similar to assessment according to density is assessment according to water content. The greater the percentage of water the more Yin. Drying or dehydrating makes more Yang; similarly it follows that liquifying or making more watery makes more Yin. This is an important consideration when selecting, preparing, and cooking food.

Colour. In the solar spectrum the colours are classified from Red (Yang) to Violet (Yin). The longer the wave length the more Yang.

Here we should draw special attention to an important difference between the vegetable kingdom and the animal kingdom. The vegetable kingdom is characterized by chlorophyll, the life-blood of plants, which is green and represents a Yin class of life in relation to the animal kingdom which is characterized by haemoglobin, red blood, Yang.

Pigmentation of parts of the body serves as a good indicator of a Yin or Yang constitution or condition. Auburn hair is classified as very Yang; blonde hair, Yang; black hair, Yin: and hair that is grey or white is far too Yin. As regards colour of the skin there is a difference between redness on account of pigmentation and redness due to presence of excess blood from over-dilation of subcutaneous capillaries. Pigmentation and the shape of the fingernails are good indicators of the state of health.

To make a diagnosis an acupuncture therapist, in addition to reading the pulses and noting breathing rate and depth, will take note of a whole host of items such as we have just indicated.

Since proper energy or Yin/Yang balance means health, an imbalance indicates something needs attention. The chief concern of the acupuncturist is to assess *to what extent* the flow of life energy is out of normal or proper balance. He also wants to know location and causes of the imbalance before deciding what to do about it. He knows that nature has an incredible power of self-adjustment and of self-harmonization. In an ordinarily healthy person this self-adjustment and harmonization is going on all the time. If for one reason or another an imbalance has occurred and has not adjusted itself but *is detected soon enough* only a very slight 'push in the right direction' suffices to restore balance and harmony.

The really skilled therapist prevents serious illness by discovering the first signs and dealing with those: but before we go on to describe his diagnostic methods more fully we need to have some sort of appreciation and understanding of how he visualizes the life-energy flow through man; that is, the flow Heaven to Earth and Earth to Heaven.

CHAPTER FOUR

LIFE-ENERGY PATHWAYS

Although Life-energy (vital-force) permeates every living cell and tissue throughout the entire organism there is, according to Chinese tradition, a rhythmic circulation of this life-energy within the human body along quite clearly demarcated pathways. Twelve of these, known as the twelve organ meridians, run just under the skin. Each is linked with an inner organ, the meridian being named after the organ with which it is directly linked and associated.

On these meridians there are points at which the energy flow can be controlled, and the organ or function connected with it affected. The points at which action can be taken are known as *acupuncture points.* On the twelve organ meridians there are over 300 acupuncture points on each side of the body. In addition to the twelve organ meridians, which are bilateral, there are two special meridians, one on the centre line of the front of the body, and onc on the centre line of the back. On these two there are in all fifty-two points.

That is by no means all: there are also special well known, and some jealously guarded secret points, that are not on any of the meridians. We can reckon, then, that altogether there are at least eight hundred points at which the life-energy can be influenced.

Although we may know these points as *acupuncture* points, and acupuncture means literally 'pricking with a needle', they are *not all* treatable with a needle. Because of the position of some points, a needle is unsuitable or dangerous if not located with sufficient accuracy. Some points are forbidden to the needle because treatment with a needle at the point is dangerous. As an example, a needle inserted at a point known as 'blue death' causes death by stopping the heart action. This point is *strictly* forbidden to the needle, and, as with other points forbidden to needle, alternative methods of treatment must be used. We shall be discussing these later on.

The illustration shows the paths of the twelve bilateral organ meridians and the two median paths. Although these meridians are shown on one side of the body it must be realized that they occur on both – left and right. The diagram shows the general line of flow: some of these lines, paths, or *streams* begin at the finger tips and end on the face; some begin on the face and end at the toes; some begin at the toes and end on the thorax; some begin on the thorax and end at the finger tips. The ending of one line is connected by a linking inner pathway to the beginning of the next; thus there is no break in circulation continuity.

Six of the twelve organs are known as Yang organs, and the energy in their organ meridians is *Yang energy*. Six of the twelve are called Yin organs, and their energy is *Yin energy*.

Yang energy is also known as 'Breath of Heaven' and Yin as 'Breath of Earth'. How this shows itself in the meridian flow is illustrated by imagining a

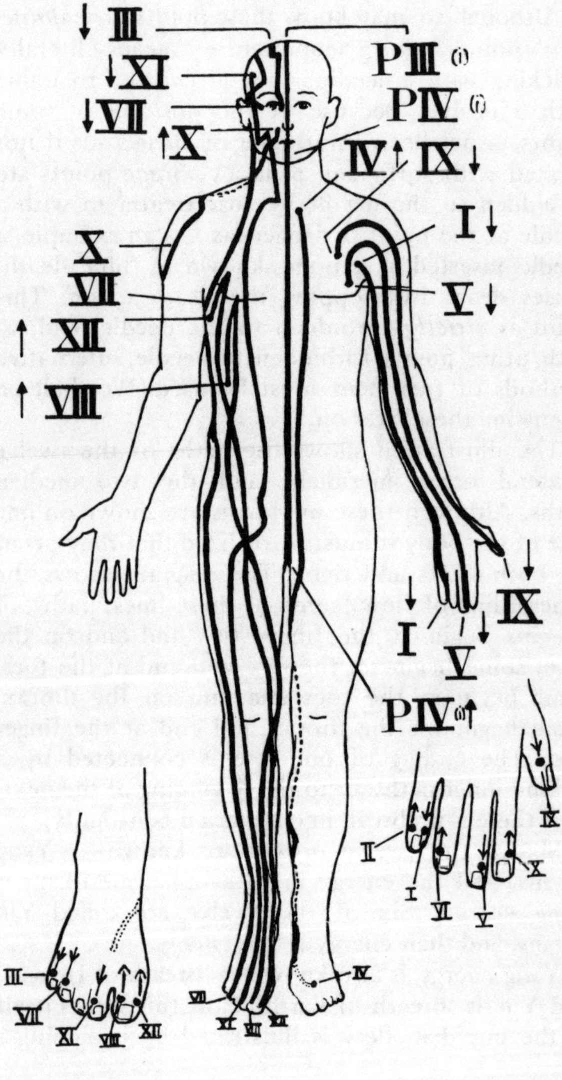
III
XI
VII
X
PIII (i)
PIV (i)
IV
IX
I
X
VII
V
XII
VIII
IX
I
V
PIV (i)
IX
II
X
I
VI
V
IV
III
VII
XI
VIII
XII
VII
XI
VIII
XII

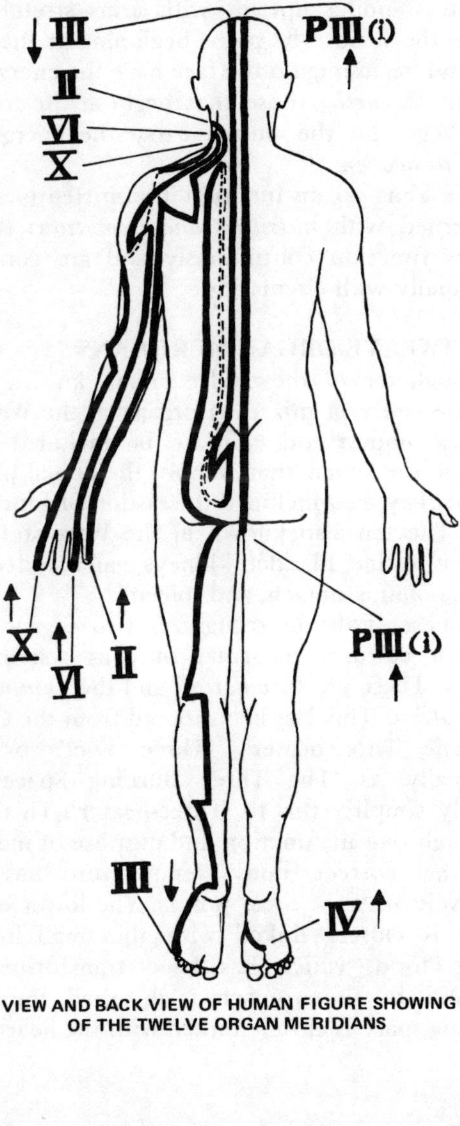

FRONT VIEW AND BACK VIEW OF HUMAN FIGURE SHOWING PATHS OF THE TWELVE ORGAN MERIDIANS

person standing upright with arms stretched up above the head. The paths beginning at the finger tips and beginning on the face have the energy flow *heaven to earth*: those that begin at the toes and that begin on the thorax carry the energy flow *earth to heaven.*

The Yang organs function intermittently and are concerned with *nutrition and excretion*: the Yin organs function continuously and are concerned principally with circulation.

THE TWELVE ORGAN MERIDIANS

Although ten of the twelve organs known to the Chinese are recognized as organs in the West, the Chinese understood *more* to be included in the idea of the organ than simply the actual physical organ; they also included the notion of function as well. The ten also known in the West are: heart, small intestine, bladder, kidneys, gall bladder, liver, lungs, colon, stomach, and spleen.

Chinese tradition recognizes two organs which western cultures recognize only as systems, not organs. These are *Circulation* and the *Temperature Regulation.* This last is translated from the Chinese as 'The Three-heater', 'Three Foci', or more poetically as 'The Three Burning Spaces': we usually simplify this to 'Three-heater'. This organ, although *one* in function and purpose of maintaining the correct body temperature has *three* relatively distinct focal points. The lower burning space is closely linked with the small intestine where food, which has been transformed and prepared by the stomach, is absorbed; the middle burning space is closely linked with the heart as the distributor of blood which has passed through and been prepared by the lungs; finally the upper burning space is linked with the area of the Circle of Willis where the comparison is made between the temperature of the world outside the body and that within the body. The information is provided at this area by the temperature of the air breathed in and the temperature of the blood stream in an artery; the information being transmitted through the nerve system to the brain.

In addition to the twelve organ meridians there are special linkages of points on several organ meridians. These form what are, in effect, regulatory reservoirs of energy. There are specific acupuncture points for controlling these reservoirs. Properly used, these points (eight in all) in a single treatment can have truly dynamic results upon conditions which western medicine is scarcely able to treat at all. Among other conditions the acupuncturist will take action at these special points to restore correct hormone balance.

We, in the West, tend to learn each acupuncture point as a number rather than by name. Nevertheless some of the traditional names for the points give valuable clues to the usefulness of the point. For example: the fourth point on the Large intestine meridian has the special name 'The Great Eliminator'. Although this point is on the hand, between thumb and first finger, it is one of the most powerful of all points for dealing, not only with the constipation and diarrhoea, but also with practically *any* faults of the eliminatory function anywhere on the body or in the body, as well as with a great many symptoms which result from faulty elimination. The first point on this same meridian is known as the 'Dentists' point'. One would expect a point with a name like that to be suitable for use anaesthetically during tooth extraction or other dental operations. It is so used, and we have had practical experience of its use in this way. But this point is by no means limited to dentists' requirements, it has special significance in a form of treatment known as the Five Elements method.

There are, for example, two points on the abdomen with names which, as it were, speak for themselves: the 'Sea of Energy' and the 'Harmonizer'. At the first of these a vast reservoir of stored energy can be released into the system or dammed up if it is escaping too rapidly into the system. The Harmonizer is a great point for balancing out conflicts and tensions, physical and emotional.

CHAPTER FIVE

THE INDIVIDUAL MERIDIANS

Without going into details that could only be of interest to a therapist or student of acupuncture, we very briefly trace the paths of the individual meridians. It should always be borne in mind that the meridians are bilateral, that is to say, they occur on both sides, left and right.

ENERGY PATHS

The **HEART** meridian begins in the armpit and goes down the arm, forearm and hand to finish at the root of the little finger nail. This meridian has *nine points.*

The **SMALL INTESTINE** meridian has its first point on the little finger at the root of the fingernail; the path travels up the forearm and arm, over the shoulder, up the neck to the face, just in front of the ear. There are *nineteen points* on this meridian.

The **BLADDER** meridian has its first point at either side of the nose at the inner corner of the eye. The path goes over the forehead and head, down the back, back of the thighs and legs, along the outer border of the foot to finish at the root of the little toenail. There are *sixty-seven points* on this meridian.

The **KIDNEYS** meridian has its first point on the sole of the foot, from whence it travels up the inner side of the leg and thigh, over the abdomen and chest to finish just below the collar-bone. There are *twenty-seven points* on this meridian.

The **CIRCULATION** meridian (by some acupuncturists this is called the **HEART CONSTRICTOR** or **HEART SURROUND**) begins on the breast, goes to and down the arm and forearm, over the palm of the hand to finish at the root of the middle fingernail. There are *nine points* on this meridian. It has the distinguishing feature that on this meridian there are no forbidden points. Any of them may be treated with a needle, moxa, or massage. All the other meridians have points forbidden to one form of treatment or another.

The **THREE-HEATER** meridian begins at the root of the nail of the ring finger, the path going over the back of the hand, up the forearm and arm, over the back of the shoulder, up the side of the neck, round over the ear to the outer tip of the eyebrow, where it ends at its *twenty-third point.*

The **GALL BLADDER** meridian starts near the outer corner of the eye from where it goes back and forth over the skull and nape of the neck, forward over the shoulder, down the side of the chest, abdomen, thighs and legs to finish at the root of the fourth toe nail. There are *forty-four points* on this meridian.

The **LIVER** meridian begins near the big toe nail and goes up over the foot to the inner side of the leg and thigh, over the abdomen to just below the ribs, where it finishes at the *fourteenth point.*

The **LUNGS** meridian begins on the side of the chest, curving round the armpit it then goes down the arm and forearm to finish near the thumbnail. There are *eleven points* on this meridian.

The **COLON** or **LARGE INTESTINE** meridian has its first point at the root of the nail of the forefinger from where it goes up the first finger to and over the wrist, up the arm, over the shoulder and neck, finishing on the face close to the nostril. This meridian has *eleven points.*

The **STOMACH** meridian begins just below the eye; the path travels down the face and neck, over the front of the chest and abdomen, down the thigh and leg to finish at the root of the second toe nail, at the *forty-fifth point.*

The **SPLEEN** meridian begins at the big toe nail and travels up the inner side of the foot, leg, and thigh, over the abdomen and chest as far as a point between the sixth and seventh rib where it finishes. There are *twenty-one points* on this meridian.

TWO CENTRE-LINE MERIDIANS

In addition to these twelve bilateral meridians there are the two centre-line meridians known as the **CONCEPTION** and **GOVERNOR** Vessels.

The **GOVERNOR** vessel begins at the tip of the coccyx and goes up the centre line of the spine, over the skull and face to finish in the centre of the upper gum between the roots of the two front teeth. This vessel has *twenty-seven points.*

The **CONCEPTION** vessel also begins not far from the tip of the spine, but this one travels up the front mid-line to finish at the centre of the lower lip at the *twenty-fourth point.*

So far we have talked about paths along which vital energy flows; but we have not said whether there is in scientific fact any anatomical justification for the meridians being mapped as they are, and for the points being so exactly placed. How the ancients knew where these points were, and knew so exactly, we may perhaps never discover; but what we can do is to look into any modern apparent confirmation of the existence of the meridians and points. This we shall now do by briefly giving an account of the discoveries of Professor Kim Bong Han.

CHAPTER SIX

KIM BONG HAN

In the Far East in spite of well over one hundred years of western medicine propaganda and the setting up of western medicine hospitals, Western and Eastern medicine remained poles apart. Sad to say, those who belonged to the western schools tended to adopt a supercilious attitude of superiority towards native practitioners. Fortunately a sensible and courageous step was taken by the appropriate authorities of the Democratic Peoples' Republic of Korea, who set up and financed a research team to enquire into acupuncture.

OFFICAL ENCOURAGEMENT

The research team, led by Professor Kim Bong Han, was provided with adequate funds, all requisite modern instruments and equipment and, above all, given official encouragement throughout long years of hard work, difficulties and frustrations. The outcome has been the publication of (1) a report delivered by Professor Kim Bong Han at a Scientific Symposium at Pyongyang, November 30, 1963; (2) two Papers read by him at the first Scientific Symposium of the Korean Society of Kyungrak held in Pyongyang on April 15, 1965. These Papers detail discoveries of such importance to biology and medical science that more than one of the generally accepted theories and prevailing notions may have to be completely re-assessed.

Whenever we have mentioned Kim Bong Han's discoveries to medical doctors over here in the West, we have met with the immediate reaction, 'Have his discoveries been confirmed?' To which we have to answer that, as far as we are at present aware, no other scientific investigators have confirmed Bong Han's discoveries – but note that a discovery is not invalidated simply by not having been confirmed. Confirmation is unlikely until a body of scientific research workers has been adequately financed for a long enough period; the work is quite beyond the resources of a private individual.

We are therefore prepared tentatively to accept the validity of the Bong Han discoveries on the grounds that the Professor and the members of the team he led are neither liars nor lunatics, but highly intelligent and gifted scientists who have discovered facts important enough to have been considered worth publishing in several languages by the Medical Science Press, Pyongyang, Korea.

TWO MAJOR ACCOMPLISHMENTS

The two major accomplishments of the Bong Han team are:

1. Demonstrating the existence of the independent functional-morphological system known traditionally, in Korean, as the Kyungrak system. It is experimentally verified that at traditional acupuncture points (known in Korean medicine as Khyunghyul positions) there exists a hitherto unknown and unsuspected structure now named a Bonghan Corpuscle; and, linking the corpuscles, there is a system of ducts through which a

fluid circulates – the ducts follow traditional meridian paths.

2. Discovery of unique granules (named Bonghan Sanal) which circulate in the Kyungrak system and grow into new cells; the old cells of organs and tissues disintegrate and turn into Sanal while moving through the Kyungrak system. Thus an incessant renewal or self-renovation takes place in the acupuncture meridian system.

Korea is not the only country to have made significant advances in medicine. A small pamphlet on *Acupuncture Anaesthesia* (published by the Foreign Languages Press, Peking 1972) printed in the People's Republic of China shows how China's medical and scientific workers have re-discovered acupuncture anaesthesia by applying modern scientific knowledge and methods to traditional Chinese medicine. Films made in China about acupuncture anaesthesia have already had sufficiently wide showing in the West, so that now it is the few who are unaware, unlike ten or twelve years ago, when only a few English-speaking people had ever heard of acupuncture.

Having briefly described the Life Force concept and the paths of Flow, we now have to turn our attention to the ways in which the traditional acupuncturist finds out what is wrong, where the energy flow is unbalanced, or the regulator system has broken down.

CHAPTER SEVEN

DIAGNOSIS

Thousands of years before the Christian era the Chinese recognized that there was a relationship between heartbeat, respiration rate and blood flow: and that this relationship reflected the state of health of the organism as a whole. This is acknowledged in Western medicine, indeed it is an essential part of clinical examination to note the patient's breathing rate, whether deep or shallow, steady or irregular, easy or laboured, and how many heartbeats to one breath.

When, in the West, one talks about 'taking the patient's pulse', one's mind immediately goes to the wrist where the radial artery is easily felt pulsating. There are several other places where the pulsations could as easily be felt – wherever an artery runs close to a bone and near to the surface.

The truly great discovery made by the Chinese was that through the *pulses* it is possible to read, not merely the general state of health of the organism as a whole, but also the health of each inner organ separately. Has the organ much or little energy? Is it congested? Is the energy escaping or is there too little? Is the energy over-active or under-active? Are the polar changes happening as they should?

They soon discovered that at the wrist there are twelve distinctly discernible pulses. That is to say: on each wrist there are three positions, and at each

FEELING ONE'S OWN PULSES FEELING THE PULSES OF A PATIENT

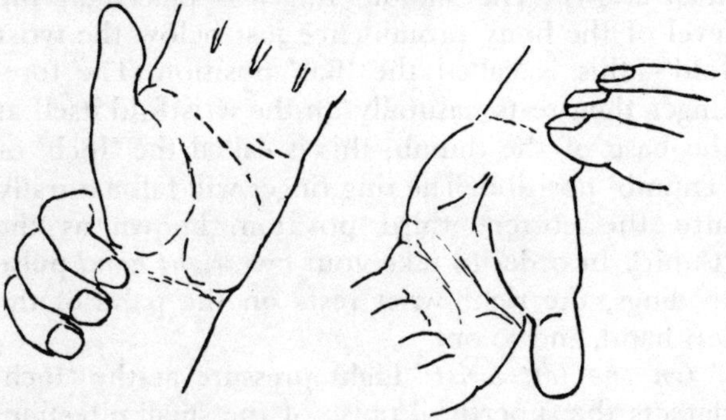

THE RADIAL PULSES POSITIONS

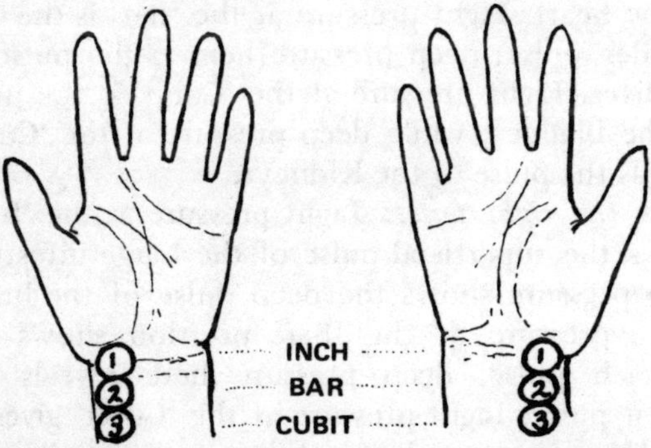

position there are two depths. At each of these twelve 'pulses' the inner state of a different organ is reflected.

HOW TO TAKE PULSE READINGS

In order to take your own *left hand* pulse readings, sit relaxed with the back of the left wrist resting on the palm of the right hand, curling the fingers over so that the tips rest on the radial artery (*see illustration*). The middle finger is placed at the level of the bony prominence just below the wrist fold – this is called the 'Bar' position. The fore-finger then rests naturally *on* the wristfold itself at the base of the thumb, this is called the 'Inch' or 'Thumb' position. The ring finger will fall naturally into the correct third position, known as the 'Cubit'. In order to take your own *right hand* pulse readings, the right wrist rests on the palm of the left hand, and so on.

On the left wrist: Light pressure at the 'Inch' detects the superficial pulse of the small intestine: deep pressure reveals the deep pulse, which is that of the heart. Light pressure at the 'Bar' is the Gall Bladder pulse; deep pressure here is the pulse of the liver. Light pressure at the 'Cubit' is the pulse of the bladder; while deep pressure at the 'Cubit' reveals the pulse of the Kidneys.

On the right wrist: Light pressure at the 'Inch' shows the superficial pulse of the Large intestine: deep pressure shows the deep pulse of the lungs. Light pressure at the 'Bar' position shows the stomach pulse, deep pressure here reveals the spleen pulse. Light pressure at the 'Cubit' gives us the Three-heater pulse, and deep pressure gives the Circulation pulse.

Almost anyone, after a very little practice, can detect differences at these pulse positions: but it takes a long time and a great deal of practice to become proficient in reading and interpreting the pulses. If, for example, one of the pulses is scarcely discernible, this does not necessarily indicate a weakness, deficiency or disturbance. Quite the contrary, it could well indicate that, at *that hour* of the day, at *that season* of the year, at *that phase* of the moon, and in relation to other circumstances, the pulse is as it should be.

THE ORIENTAL PRACTITIONER

When feeling the pulses the oriental practitioner 'listens' to them much as one listens to an orchestra – each pulse representing one of the instrumentalists. Taken all together the melody should be a happy and harmonious one. It is as if one is listening to that person's Life-song. If the melody is not joyous and harmonious at least one of the players is out of tune or out of time. The practitioner has to locate the discordant player. The practitioner has an almost ritual approach to the pulses; this has so often been sneered at by westerners who understand so little of Far Eastern wisdom.

The oriental doctor is quite unperturbed if it takes a whole hour to read, re-read and assess the pulses, and generally examine the patient in order to make his diagnosis. He knows that if this hour of diagnosis is followed by thirty seconds of treatment at the right place, more good will be done for the patient than if thirty seconds snappy guesswork diagnosis is followed by an hour of dubious treatment or a prescription for a bottle of drug pills.

What is the Life Force doing in each organ and in each organ-meridian? Is there so little vital energy that it speaks in the pulse as if it were a thin drawn silk thread? Is the energy hurriedly pouring itself away as if the sands were rapidly running out? Is there somewhere a blockage against which the Life Force is striving to push its way? Is the life-effort erratic?

SECRETS REVEALED

The human being will, through the pulses, reveal the innermost secrets of the Life Force animating it, and the message will be truthful. Life always speaks truth about itself – one simply has to learn at what level to listen. The practitioner listens with open mind and sympathetic heart. He accepts the message as the Life Force in the patient gives it.

There are many methods, other than the pulses, for finding out what is wrong with a patient. For example there is the method known as Abdominal Diagnosis. Using this method alone the skilled (specialist) practitioner is able to learn all that it is necessary to know about the patient by a sensitive palpation of the abdomen.

The practitioner, of course, will listen to *whatever* the patient has to say about his aches or pains, about his domestic or social difficulties and problems, his hopes, fears, joys and sorrows, what he eats and what he drinks; he listens to everything because in amongst all the items there may be some quite important clue to help in building up the general picture so that the key factors can be located.

Having made a thorough examination and arrived at a clear diagnosis, the practitioner then decides at which acupuncture point or points to take action, and what kind of action to take.

CHAPTER EIGHT

WHERE AND HOW

Quite early on we indicated that the two polarities of energy, 'Breath of Heaven' (Yang) and 'Breath of Earth' (Yin) change polarity from one to the other in regular rhythm.

In the Organ Meridian system the energy flowing from the thorax to the fingertip is **YIN** predominant energy: as the energy approaches the extremity the polarity begins to change and, by the time the tip of the finger is reached, **YIN** dominance is extinguished and with the flow beginning from the finger tip towards the body, **YANG** dominance begins.

In the central area, i.e., head and chest, even though the energy flows from one meridian to another, there is no polarity change. It is not until the energy begins to approach the other extremity that polarity change begins. **YANG** dominance is extinguished at the toes and **YIN** dominance begins again with the upward meridian flow.

The polarity change is not sudden, but happens gradually between elbow and finger tips and between knee and toes.

There is a principle, well known in Judo, that a person's balance can be most easily upset at the moment his weight is being shifted from one foot to the other. This principle applies in acupuncture, and the vital energy flow can be most easily retarded or accelerated at points where the energy

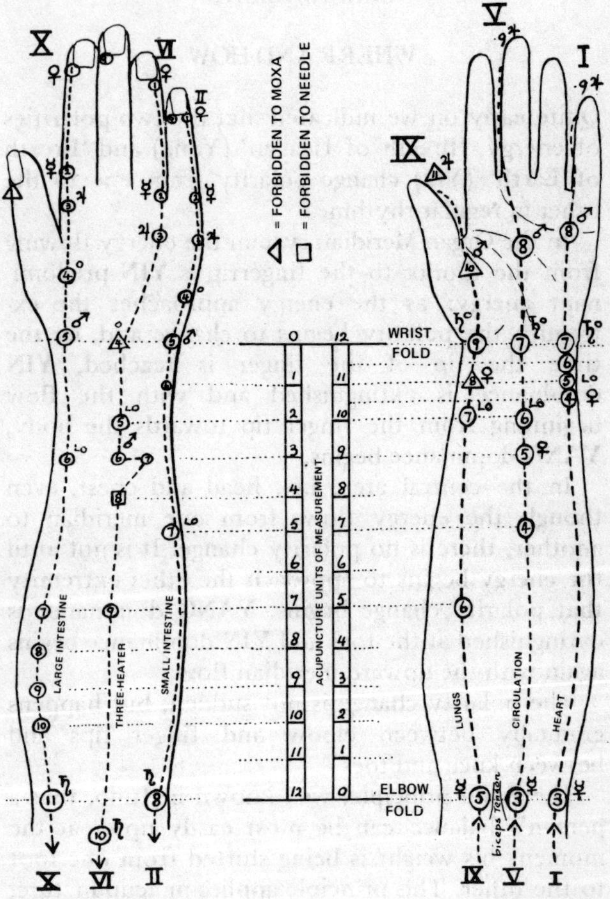

= FORBIDDEN TO MOXA
= FORBIDDEN TO NEEDLE
WRIST FOLD
ELBOW FOLD
ACUPUNCTURE UNITS OF MEASUREMENT
LARGE INTESTINE
THREE-HEATER
SMALL INTESTINE
LUNGS
CIRCULATION
HEART
biceps Tendon
X
VI
II
IX
V
I

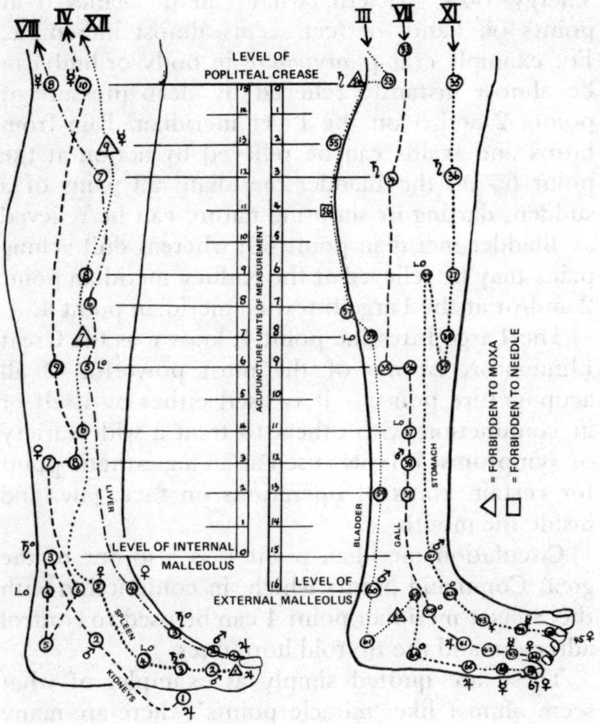
VIII
IV
XII
III
VII
XI
LEVEL OF
POPLITEAL CREASE
ACUPUNCTURE UNITS OF MEASUREMENT
LEVEL OF INTERNAL
MALLEOLUS
LEVEL OF
EXTERNAL MALLEOLUS
LIVER
SPLEEN
KIDNEYS
BLADDER
GALL
STOMACH
= FORBIDDEN TO MOXA
= FORBIDDEN TO NEEDLE

is changing polarity. It is therefore at acupuncture points below the knee and below the elbow that the most important Control or Master and Command points will be found.

To any Westerner unaccustomed to the oriental 'energy flow' pattern, what can be achieved at points on hands or feet seems almost incredible. For example cramp *anywhere* in body or limb can be almost instantly relieved by deep pressure at points 2 and 3 on the Liver meridian. Pain from burns and scalds can be relieved by action at the point 65 on the Bladder meridian: all pains of a sudden, darting or shooting nature can be relieved at Bladder meridian point 60; whereas dull aching pains may be relieved at the Kidney meridian point 2 and/or at the Large Intestine meridian point 4.

The Large Intestine point 4, known as the Great Eliminator, is one of the most powerful of all acupuncture points – it is used either by itself or in conjunction with others to treat a wide variety of symptoms; it is also used as an anaesthetic point for certain kinds of operations on face, jaw, and inside the mouth.

Circulation meridian point 6 is also one of the great Command points which, in conjunction with the Spleen meridian point 4 can be used to control adrenalin and the thyroid hormones.

These are quoted simply as examples of what seem almost like 'miracle points': there are many such.

Partly what makes them seem so miraculous is because so often only one needle will be used to bring about dramatic and spectacular results. According to tradition, no more needles than are absolutely *necessary* should be used. Inserting a number of needles to impress the patient and to help him feel that he is getting his money's worth is looked upon as quite contemptible quackery by the traditional Chinese practitioner. Not only is it not sensible to use several points when one would do, it is also bad practice because, far from adding to the therapeutic effect, the extra needles could drain away and waste the patient's vital force. A true master of acupuncture will diagnose with such care that, more often than not, he will be able to select one point only for treatment.

Having selected the acupuncture point at which the practitioner considers action should be taken, he will do whatever is appropriate, using one of the three principal techniques: Needle, Moxa, or Massage.

NEEDLE TECHNIQUE

In ancient times needles of flint and bone, even thorns, were used before the various metals gold, silver, steel and copper were introduced. Nowadays, although one may hear of occasional use of gold or silver needles, those most generally used are made of very fine steel, wound for a third of their length with fine copper wire forming the handle. The use of the copper is not merely to make a handle but the *copper and the steel* generate a minute electric current, the direction of flow being dependent on whether the steel is warmer than the copper, or vice versa.

Even though a needle may be three inches long, or even twice that, it is rarely inserted more than a few millimetres. The acupuncture points (or Bong

Han Corpuscles) are mostly only just under the surface of the skin. The therapeutic effect does not so much depend upon the depth to which the needle is inserted as upon *how* it is inserted and *what* is done with it once it is in.

Is it put in quickly and removed slowly? Is it held still all the time it is in? Is it held at all after insertion? Is it twiddled, turned, vibrated up and down, or shaken from side to side? Is it left in for a set period? Is it inserted while the patient is breathing in or out? The practitioner has to know exactly what difference each variation will make. This knowledge cannot be acquired in half-an-hour; but takes years of study.

We now quote a page from the *Nei Ching* as an example of the quaint language in which Ch'i Po explained to the Emperor the laws and methods used. This passage begins, of course, with the need to observe the Laws of Nature:

> All the laws of acupuncture must attend upon the sun, the moon, the planets, the stars, and the four seasons. These are the eight factors of the atmosphere, and when the atmosphere is established one can apply acupuncture.
>
> Thus when the weather is warm and the sun clear and bright, the blood of man flows gently and his secretions protect his breath (vigour) and keep it volatile. Hence the blood flows easily and the breath moves smoothly. When the weather is cold and the sun is darkened, man's blood coagulates and does not flow, and his hitherto protected breath sinks low and perishes.
>
> When the moon begins to wax, then blood and breath come to life, the essences receive new incentive and guard the breath of life which begins to be active. When the moon is full to the rim, there is abundance of blood and breath (within man), the muscles and the flesh are

firm and strong. When the moon is empty to the rim, the muscles and the flesh become reduced, the arteries and the veins become empty, and the hitherto guarded breath departs, leaving the body in a deserted condition. Therefore one should act in accordance with the weather and the seasons in order to have blood and breath thoroughly adjusted and harmonized – and consequently – when the weather is cold one should not apply acupuncture. But when the day is warm there should not be any hesitation about the advisability of acupuncture. (from *Nei Ching*, book 8, chapter 26.)

Ch'i Po goes on to explain in considerable detail what the results will be if acupuncture is undertaken at the wrong time or if the wrong kind of treatment is given; he emphasizes that those who do not take into account the atmospheres to be avoided are ignorant and should not be in practice as therapists for, far from curing diseases, they cause them.

'But' he says, 'if those who are experts in medical treatment take into consideration the time of the treatment they will not inflict any hurt.'

After reading the *Nei Ching* a number of times and, as it were, getting soaked in the oriental ways of thinking and expression, the detailed instructions make sense and are in reality quite easy to follow; even though at first it may not appear all that simple, partly because of quaint and archaic language. Of the many needle methods we now quote, as an example, a few lines on the draining technique.

In order to drain one must use *fang*, the right condition or method. *Fang* means that one must apply draining when the atmospheric condition is favourable, one must apply it when the moon is full, one must apply it when

> the day is warm, and one must apply it when the body is in an orderly state. One must apply it when the breath is being inhaled. Then the needle must be inserted, and it must be repeated when the breath is being inhaled again. But the needle must be turned around, and this must be repeated when the breath is being exhaled; and then the needle must be slowly drawn out.

What is so charming and delightful about this medical treatise is that the Emperor is recorded as always being so very appreciative of whatever Ch'i Po tells him:

> 'How wonderful this reasoning! To bring into agreement man's body with Yin and Yang, the two principles in nature, and with the four seasons; his echoing of want and fullness, his response to the most subtle influences; who but you could so interpret it?'

For one reason or another action with a needle is forbidden at some points, therefore if the point that has to be treated happens to be one that is forbidden to the needle a different method of treatment has to be used. The alternatives are usually either Moxa or Massage. Unless the point is specifically forbidden to moxa, moxa may be used on any point. No points are specifically forbidden to massage.

MOXA TECHNIQUE

This is a method of applying heat by burning a small cone of artemisia (dried leaves of the mugwort) over the point. The burning cone must not be allowed to burn the patient, but must be removed at the last moment when it is felt as too hot. Experiments have been made over several thousand years to find other effective ways of applying heat to the acupuncture points; but nothing has so far been discovered to equal the effect of the dried artemisia.

Moxa is often used as a method of preference, according to the practitioner's choice. Sometimes moxa has to be used instead of a needle during certain periods or in certain places as, for example, when the use of needles is restricted during certain phases of pregnancy.

There are times when neither needle nor moxa should be used as, for example, on children below certain ages. In these cases a special kind of massage is given at an acupuncture point. Ten or fifteen seconds of the appropriate massage will bring about just as miraculous a result as needles or moxa.

Nowadays experiments are still going on, and new methods are being tried; methods that were quite unknown to the ancients, as for example, electrical stimulation at acupuncture points. Especially do we notice new techniques being tried out in the development of the anaesthetic use of acupuncture.

Acupuncture, in the widest sense of the term, shows signs of being the 'therapy of the future'. In its widest sense acupuncture must be understood to include preventive as well as therapeutic measures, and thus will include such important aspects as diet.

This is not simply wishful thinking, but from our own contact with people and with therapists (including the ordinary western medical practitioner) we see and hear definite signs that more and more therapists are *actually wanting to heal* their patients because they are human beings in need, and not merely treating them as a 'fee': at the same time more and more people want to have their aches and pains *healed*, not merely covered up or shifted elsewhere. There seems to be an increasing number of people interested in how to avoid illness altogether, rather than in how to get better once the illness has struck. By this we are, of course, not referring to the various vaccinations and inoculations against this or that. Real preventive treatment amounts to living sensibly in proper harmony with nature. We shall now discuss this aspect.

CHAPTER NINE

NOT ALL NEEDLES

Over and over again in the *Nei Ching* we read the injunction to live 'in proper harmony with nature'.

The Yellow Emperor, in his days, seemed to have quite a lot of trouble with his subjects who were not living in proper harmony with nature, and had not been doing so for some time. He was a thoroughly practical man, and did not shut his eyes to the reality of the situation. He recognized that there were two goals to hold constantly in mind, and that these had to be aimed for simultaneously.

First there was the relatively short-term goal or policy which was that, having recognized that people were already sick, he had to do something about treating the actual diseases and sicknesses rife at that time.

Secondly it was necessary to work towards the long-term goal of having an established healthy community. This required a policy of foresight and prevention that would keep a healthy people in a state of health.

If it was important to bear these two objectives in mind in the old days, how much more important is it to do likewise today when such a wide range of diseases flourish and increase alarmingly!

The Yellow Emperor's precepts are as valid now as they were then, and we make no apologies for repeating them in order to drive home an awareness of *urgency* today.

Whether we like to think of the rulers being sages, or the sages being the rulers, the fact remains that those who ruled over the people did so in a far wider sense than the purely politically administrative sense. *Wise men* ruled over the people politically, economically, culturally, and regulated the health of the people. In the *Nei Ching* we read:

> . . . the sages did not treat those who were already ill; they instructed those who were not yet ill. They did not want to rule those who were already rebellious; they guided those who were not yet rebellious. To administer medicines to diseases which have already developed and to suppress revolts which have already developed is comparable to the behaviour of those persons who begin to dig a well after they have become thirsty, and of those who begin to cast weapons after they have already engaged in battle.

If the sages did not treat the sick, who did?

It became the task of the physicians, trained in the general principles of the sages, to do something practical about dealing adequately with rebels (i.e., the sick). Not in the sense of punishing wrongdoers, the illness itself representing the merited punishment, but rather giving them *corrective* treatment to set them back on the right path of obedience and health. This represents a very different orientation from that of the physician whose aim is to alleviate pain using any means that will get rid of the pain regardless of long term consequences or side-effects; or one who prescribes drugs to cover up, conceal, or transfer discomforts and unsightliness regardless of long-term effects.

We now come across what is perhaps one of the most important of all medicine-philosophy principles – and one which, alas, seems utterly disregarded at the present day in almost every corner of the globe. Here we quote again from the *Nei Ching*:

> A healthy and well-balanced person is not affected by disease. Those who are habitually without disease help to train and to adjust those who are sick, for *those who treat should be free from illness.* Therefore they train the patient to adjust his breathing, and *in order to train the patient, they act as example.*

How often at the present day are we able to see medical practitioners themselves fit enough to act as examples to their patients?

The breathing rate of the patient should be compared with that of the doctor; the patient's pulse rate with that of the doctor. It could be said that nowadays this is not necessary because every doctor has a watch by which to time the patient's breathing and pulse rate whereas in ancient times there were no watches. To this we answer: Ownership of a watch is *not* a valid excuse for ill or indifferent health.

In these days of addictive drugs and surgery one of the most neglected ways of looking after one's health is *proper feeding habits.* To us it seems obvious common sense to say that you should not eat unless you are hungry; but many people eat regularly at a certain time out of habit, certainly not on account of hunger. Also, people tend to eat far too much and, of course, very often unsuitable foods.

DIETETIC PRINCIPLES

Prescribing a particular diet for someone who needs to slim, or who has diabetic troubles, thyroid imbalances, over-acidity, under-acidity, etc., is relatively unimportant and only scratching at the surface of the problem of correct diet. Attention should be seriously paid to a thorough assimilation of dietetic *principles*, so that each individual is able to choose according to his or her own constitutional make-up, needs, means, environment, and according to foods available.

The Yellow Emperor attached very great importance to correct diet. Quite a lot of attention is given to diet in the *Nei Ching*. Traditionally all foods are considered as coming into one or another of five categories or flavours. He talks of the five flavours to mean the five basic and representative types of food, namely: bitter, sour, sweet, pungent, and salty. In the *Nei Ching* it is affirmed 'nothing excels the deliciousness of these five flavours. Human desires are not alike, therefore everyone has at his disposal all of them'.

> If people pay attention to the five flavours and mix them well, their bones will remain straight, their muscles will remain tender and young, their breath and blood will circulate freely, their pores will be fine in texture, and consequently, their breath and bones will be filled with the essence of life. If, furthermore, the people carefully follow the Right Way as though it were a law, theirs will be a long life.

Two points from this quotation need further explanation: first the assertion that everyone has at his disposal all of them. It should be noted that all five are not necessarily available in equal quantities – the proportions will depend upon the climate or part of the world one is living in. The differences in proportion are due to nature's law: that which belongs in a particular climate is produced by that climate. Expressed in terms of

Yang and Yin: Yang produces Yin; Yin produces Yang.

The second point is that of 'mixing well'. In the old days of Huang Ti and earlier the people were taught how to arrive at the best balance in the diet while, at the same time, retaining considerable freedom of individual choice. In other words, a diet does not have to be monotonous simply because it is well balanced.

It is often easier to understand a point if an extreme case is quoted – even if extremes do not actually exist in such simple form.

CLIMATE AND DIET

We take as our first example a *Yang* climate: that means a climate characterized by extreme heat and dryness. Needless to say, if the climate is hot and dry beyond certain limits life is hardly possible at all – as instanced in hot tropical deserts. But in hot climates, as soon as there is sufficient moisture to support life, vegetation of an extremely Yin type flourishes: *native* bird and animal life is also very Yin (this includes humans).

Human beings native to Yang (hot) climates have Yin constitutions and Yin characteristics and will therefore need a very high proportion of Yin foods for optimum health, that is, in order to preserve their Yin-ness.

The constitutionally Yin type (native of a hot or Yang climate) will indicate his constitutional Yin-ness by (among other signs) the colour of his skin. The Yin pigmentation is a protection against the sun's rays: or may be described as a filtering device which controls the amount of light and heat rays to be absorbed into the body.

There are other characteristics quite noticeable about constitutionally Yin people: they tend, for instance, to be naturally peaceful and peace-loving: culturally they tend to be both philosophic and religious.

It is a principle of universal application that provided the diet is well regulated so that people eat that which grows in or is native to their environment, in the relative proportions in which it naturally occurs, their health will be maintained.

Yang climates produce Yin diseases, thus tropical diseases seem to affect in a major way the lungs, skin and intestines, as is demonstrated in various fevers, tuberculosis, leprosy, typhoid, dysentery, cholera, etc.

If a native of a hot climate moves to a cold climate and does not adapt appropriately to the diet proper for the cold climate he will fall a ready prey to Yang *deficiency* diseases. It will be readily seen that as far as a doctor's training is concerned, one of the most essential factors is a thorough grounding in the dietetic principles. That is to say his knowledge should go a great deal deeper than *general* knowledge. The people, ideally, should have a sound general knowledge of the relationships diet/health/climate, and be able unhesitatingly to recognize Yin and Yang fruit, vegetables, grain, and meats.

Some fruits we all know well and recognize: Pineapples, melons, oranges, grapefruit, and aubergine, all of which grow naturally in a warm or hot climate and therefore rank as extremely Yin. They are therefore suitable food in warm climates but *not* for temperate and cold climates. These fruits do not grow naturally in the British Isles and do not belong to the environment. If these are eaten at all they should be taken only in very small amounts and only on rare occasions.

A cold climate is very Yin; and, since Yin produces Yang we shall find that plant life, animals, birds and fish native to cold areas will be constitutionally and characteristically Yang, requiring a high proportion of Yang foods. So long as people eat what is proper for their environment they do not get ill. If they go against nature they suffer.

The Yellow Emperor said:

> 'From earliest times the communication with Heaven has been the very foundation of life . . . good conduct is the foundation of long life. Just as the breath of the blue sky is calm, so the will and heart of those who are pure will be in peace, and the breath of Yang will be stable in those who keep themselves in harmony with nature. Even if there are noxious spirits they cannot cause injury to those who follow the laws of the seasons. Therefore the sages preserved the natural spirit and were in harmony with the breath of Heaven, and were thus in direct communication with Heaven.
>
> 'Those who fail to preserve this communication will have their nine orifices closed from the inside, and the development of their muscles and flesh will be obstructed from the outside. This then is called: "to injure one's own body and to destroy one's own force of life".
>
> 'When people are quiet and clear, their skin and flesh is closed and protected. Even a heavy storm, afflictions, or poison, cannot injure those people who live in accord with the natural order.
>
> 'Those who rebel against the basic rules of the universe sever their own roots and ruin their true selves. Those who disobey the laws of the universe will give rise

> to calamities and visitations, while those who follow the laws of the universe remain free from dangerous illness . . . Obedience to the laws of Yin and Yang means life; disobedience means death.'

We shall now give some account of modern instances of people severing their own roots and bringing all manner of diseases and afflictions upon themselves; but before we do so, here is a quotation from Doris Grant in *Dear Housewives* (Faber & Faber, 1954).

> . . . I know beyond any shadow of doubt that we hold our health in the hollow of our hands, and that our ills, both mental and physical, are brought upon us by a life-time of wrong nutrition. This is the 'theme-song' of the famous *Medical Testament* of March 1939, in which six hundred Cheshire doctors affirmed: 'that most of the ills they were called upon to attend were the result of a life-time of wrong nutrition and inferior foods'.

CHAPTER TEN

CALAMITIES AND VISITATIONS

Striking instances of what happens when a people is moved from its natural environment to an unnatural one, are given by Laurence E.D. Knights, F.R.C.S., in his Paper presented at the Third McCarrison Society Conference of June 1973. Referring to the negro population in Sierra Leone he writes:

> Conspicuous by their absence were the degenerative diseases which plague the Western World today, and which we have every reason to believe are the products of denatured food, or what passes for food, that we inflict on our long suffering bodies. Characteristically, Negro peoples on their traditional diet who have not eaten at the table of the white man, do not suffer as he does from degenerative diseases . . . peptic ulcer . . . ulcerative colitis . . . diverticular disease of the colon . . .
>
> Cancer of the colon and rectum which comprise the second commonest cause of death from cancer in man is virtually unknown among primitive peoples, as are diseases of the appendix and gall bladder which present the two commonest abdominal emergencies in the Western World.

In contrast to the health of the negro peoples as natives to a climate and environment natural to them, is the ill health of the negroes of North America who now live in a climate and environment for which they are constitutionally unsuited.

From the Yin/Yang balance viewpoint the feeding throughout Western culture is excessively Yin; in particular is this so in the U.S.A., where in a predominantly over-processed denatured diet three chief items may justly be labelled 'the three killers', namely: white sugar, white flour, and common salt.

The list of degenerative diseases caused by faulty diet and common throughout Western Culture makes grim and unpleasant reading. Towards the close of his paper Laurence Knights says,

> Among no people are the effects of the Saccharine Disease better illustrated than by the Canadian Esquimaux. In the last twenty years, the Esquimaux have been precipitated from their traditional independent nomadic life, eating the flesh of seal and caribou, with some fat but virtually no carbohydrate and certainly none refined, to become dependent state-supported people housed in settlements . . .

He paints a sorry picture of a people taken out of their natural environment to degenerate in an unnatural one, where due to faulty nutrition a once healthy people have now the rotting teeth of western culture, constipation, peptic ulcers, appendicitis and the long, long list of worse states which follow on.

NATURE'S LAWS FLOUTED

The example we have quoted is one of innumerable instances of what is happening in a major way because of the deliberate flouting of the Laws of Nature. If the Laws are gone against beyond certain limits only disaster can result.

This observation applies to Medicine: medical treatment of sick people should not go against the Laws of Nature; unfortunately it does. A glaring instance of faulty nutrition actually being encouraged by medical men is the compulsory medication of whole communities and areas by fluoridation of the drinking water.

It is recognized by doctors that consumption of excessive amounts of sugar (any white sugar is too much) rots the teeth so, instead of taking steps to reduce sugar consumption they are willing to let a whole population be compulsorily medicated by fluoridation of the drinking water.

Reasoning of this nature was foreign to the Yellow Emperor. Instead of treating a sick person in such a way as to allow him to continue his folly, the Far Eastern tradition aimed at *corrective not palliative* treatment. If an illness did happen to develop, they insisted that it must be treated in such a way that the patient is restored to a harmonious relationship within himself and with his environment.

Manipulation of the Life Force through the needles was one well recognized way of healing in accord with nature. In skilled hands the needles were, and still are today, justly called 'healing needles'; but the art of healing embraces far more than one limited technique. Healing is not all needles.